Better Sleep Sooner

How to Turn your Sleeplessness into Sleeping Bliss, Naturally

Aaron McLoughlin

ISBN 978-0-646-56010-6
Copyright © 2011 Aaron McLoughlin

All rights reserved. No part of this document may be reproduced or transmitted in any form by any means, electronic or mechanical, including photocopying, recording and transcribing, or by any information storage or retrieval system, without permission from the author.

Cover by Aaron & Wendy McLoughlin
background Art by Aleksandar Velasevic
Printed by Publish Me, New Plymouth, New Zealand
Assisted by www.publishme.co.nz

DISCLAIMER
The material in this book will enable you to apply the strategies of Better Sleep Sooner in order to improve the quality of your life. Please note that any choices you make and actions you take using this material are your own responsibility. While endeavouring to ensure that these processes are understood the author is not responsible for the choice of lifestyles, values, content or actions people make as a result of reading 'Better Sleep Sooner'. Neither is the author responsible for any consequences of the use of the material in this book by third parties.

For Wendy ♥

About the Author

In 1995 Aaron Mcloughlin was sitting in the office of his doctor while a testing machine was being re-calibrated in order to test him once again for chemical poisoning, the result of a gardening job years earlier.

While waiting for the test he confided that he was feeling deeply unhappy with the healing process and did not know how to get through it, at which point the doctor took him through a remarkably simple yet powerful process that he had been recently taught by a hypnotherapy trainer.

Being taken through this process was like stepping from a dark cold room into a bright, sunny day. The transformation was immediate and it lasted. Aaron had to know what had just happened and how he could learn this amazing technology.

This experience began Aaron's journey into the fascinating world of Hypnosis, Neuro Linguistic Programming (NLP) and the Mind-Body Connection. Aaron passionately embraced these new tools and immediately recognised the power to not only heal and transform his own life, he also recognised the potential to help others do the same.

Fascinated by the mind and its power, Aaron has developed a number of strategies that give people simple and effective ways in which they can adjust their thinking, while improving their health and their lives. Aaron's first and second books *'The Fascination Principle'* and *'Rapid Inspired Change'* incorporated *The Fascination Principle* as a core strategy, a strategy that also underlies the *Better Sleep Sooner* strategies in this book.

Contents

Forward
By Mandy Nolan Comedian, Writer & Provocateur — 1

Chapter 1
Inspiration from Insomnia — 7
Stoems - Hypno-learning — 10

Chapter 2
The Problem with 'Sleep' — 15

Chapter 3
The Fascination Principle — 21
Asthma as Teacher — 24

Chapter 4
The Power of Emotions — 31
A Powerful Key to Emotional Healing — 33
Emotional Release Techniques — 35

Chapter 5
Reframing the Sleep Process — 47

Chapter 6
The Better Sleep Sooner Strategy — 89
The Strategy. — 93

Chapter 7
Lifestyle Considerations for Better Sleep — 105
20 Simple Tips for a Better Sleep Sooner — 128

Chapter 8
Stoems for a Better Sleep Sooner — 133
Self Hypnosis Stoem for healing sleeplessness — 134
Relaxation Stoem — 142

Appendix
Better Sleep Sooner Self-Hypnosis — 149
Power-napping — 158
Emotional Freedom Technique — 161
Better Sleep Sooner Strategy - Quick Reference — 169

Forward

By Mandy Nolan
Comedian, Writer & Provocateur

Shakespeare wasn't necessarily talking about sleep anxiety when he penned Hamlet's infamous To Be or Not to Be soliloquy. 'Sleep, perchance to dream…aye there's the rub'. His hero was perplexing about his raison d'être and in the process battling to find his bearings with his own moral compass. In doing this Hamlet likens sleep to death. A place where heart-ache and a thousand natural shocks that the 'flesh is heir to' stops.

But even Hamlet can't be assured that in death that the hideous dreams of a guilty mind won't come and haunt him for eternity. Gosh, with a framework like that the poor bloke must have been an insomniac. Perhaps the entire play was just the anxiety riddled and paranoid ravings of a bloke who'd blown things way out of proportion. Perhaps Hamlet needed a hot bath, a cup of peppermint tea and a foot massage from Ophelia. He could have then drifted into the glorious sea of sleep. Instead he couldn't stop thinking about avenging his Father's murder. I guess that sort of thing would keep you awake at night.

Sleep is the act of complete surrender. When we sleep we cannot be defensive. We cannot attack. We cannot reason. We are completely vulnerable. It's the ultimate act of letting go, a daily reminder that we must relinquish the control of the conscious world for the random unknown of the unconscious. Our ability to function in the active world is dependent on the quiet nourishment we receive during our slumber.

Now when I go to bed I imagine that I am my own iPhone, and the process of slipping between the sheets is the equivalent of plugging in for a recharge. No one wants to operate a full day with a low battery. Imagine being in an important meeting and just shutting down! Sleep is like another country, a place where we commune with our disembodied thoughts and where dreams provide a Da Vinci like code for understanding our deeper selves. We need food. We need water. We need sleep.

Without sleep we die. In some very rare cases where the brain won't release chemicals needed to sleep the result is fatal. One person went 28 days without sleep and then died. All their organs shut down, and the only reprieve they got was death. (This is a great thing to think about when you are experiencing insomnia. You could terrify yourself to sleep!) The fascinating thing is that scientists can't actually say exactly why sleep is so vital to the proper functioning of the human body. Sleep is mysterious. It's the 'nothing' we require to wake up and be the 'everything' the world requires from us.

Not sleeping is hell. For years I would go to bed and wake up only a few hours later. I'd lay awake until morning, sometimes drifting into a semi-sleep state, other times I was wide awake. The longer I lay there the worse it got. I'd get up and have a bath. Or read. Other times I'd watch TV. All the time I'd be experiencing a growing anxiety about how I was going to negotiate the next day. How would I manage a full days' work? Get the kid's lunches? Drive a long distance? I started meditating. I changed my diet. I stopped having a glass of wine in the evening. I stopped panicking and started sleeping. I noticed at the time, that not sleeping was a cycle. The more I didn't sleep, the more I didn't sleep. It was like I was burning a new pathway in my brain: a set of expectations that the bedroom equalled anxiety and frustration, not relaxation and rejuvenation.

Forward   Better Sleep Sooner

It always amazes me how much we need to sleep. As a child I hated going to bed. I was one of those kids that parents had to drive in the car at 2 in the morning. They'd get me home, carry me to bed and then I'd wake up. Sleeping just seemed like a waste of time. Being alive was far too short and far too amazing to sleep through a good portion of it. I hated going to sleep as a child because I always had this sense that I was missing out. That something was happening that didn't involve me and that sleep would render me an outsider.

Did you realise that if you live to 75 and sleep 8 hours a day, then you will have slept 219,150 hours in a lifetime. That means in the average life most people sleep for 9,131.25 days. That's just over 25 years that we spend asleep. 1/3 of our lives are spent under the doona[1]. As an adult it's now the doona time I crave not the non-doona time. There is nothing more erotic than climbing into a freshly made bed with crisp white sheets and falling asleep until morning.

I have five children, so that kind of sleep hasn't happened for some time. While now I don't suffer from insomnia, I wake up to 10 times a night to tend to my baby daughter. It seems she has the same belief system

---

[1] *Doona - Australian colloquial for duvet.*

around sleep that I had as a child. I see her lying there, wanting to be asleep but unable to slip into that deep place. She hovers on the surface. This has been amazing for me. I have now found I can sleep anywhere. On the floor. In a chair. On the couch, and just the other day I fell asleep at the wheel.

Reclaim your life by reclaiming your sleep. Aaron's book will show you how to stop thinking and start sleeping. This is the only book that I hope you fall asleep reading. God knows I did.

Chapter 1

Inspiration from Insomnia

Sleeplessness can be crazy making! Lying in bed night after night looking at the ceiling and wondering 'when oh when will sleep finally take me?'. Thoughts screeching or mumbling though the corridors of the mind. Worries and anxiety, restlessness and frustration. The monotony of the endless night without peace. Or even worse... just lying there with nothing happening, just emptiness, miserable timeless emptiness.

This is sleeplessness. It can continue for weeks, months or years and it slowly takes away your energy, clarity and peace of mind. Many people begin to become so desperate that they will do anything, eat anything, drink anything just to get one night's sleep.

This was the story of my nights. I was in the middle of a very challenging illness which I was to discover later, was influenced largely by chemical poisoning and because of that I was experiencing insomnia, night after night.

The nights seemed never-ending. Lying in bed for what seemed like the entire night, fretting and worrying about sleep. Anxiety was the nightly ritual. Lying awake imagining the next day and how exhausted I would be having had no sleep. Imagining all the sleep I had missed. Horrendous anxiety feeding upon itself and generating more and more sleeplessness and intermittent feelings of depression.

The hole that I was thinking myself into night after night seemed to get deeper and deeper. Later on I realised that I was doing a thing called Meta-thinking. A process of thinking about the thoughts, about the thoughts, etc. Much like starting on an internet web page and an hour later wondering how you came to a site about something completely unrelated to your initial search.

Our minds operate in such a fascinating and astounding way that makes this process of 'getting lost down the rabbit hole' automatic. Our minds are in a constant state of 'insatiable curiosity' which, like a child in a toy store, can grab our attention and take us for an exhausting ride that often has no real meaning or useful outcome.

It was during one of these restless, sleepless nights, out of my mind with anxiety and exhaustion and believing once again that sleep was truly beyond my reach, that a miracle occurred. In a flash of insight I realised that sleep, or getting to sleep was not the problem. Instead, I realised that it was my thinking process that was the major hurdle. In that instant my perception of lying in bed changed forever, and with that my ability to fall into sleep.

The next morning I woke up and realised that I had indeed drifted into a deep and blissful sleep. I felt refreshed and relieved, however I forgot what it was that had created the miracle. From that miraculous night onward I was falling into blissful sleep and yet I did not really know what I was doing to create this miracle. The new strategy had worked so well that it had become an unconscious program, literally invisible to my conscious mind.

It was many years later after training in Clinical Hypnotherapy and Neuro-Linguistic-Programming (NLP) that I was able to trace the unconscious path of this amazing strategy and make sense of it, and more importantly, understand its power and potential for others.

The *Better Sleep Sooner* strategy is not rocket science, it is pure simplicity. I have 'shaved' away the extraneous 'stuff' to get to the bones, which makes this system easy to learn and very difficult to forget.

The system utilises many powerful frameworks from NLP and Hypnosis while of course engaging the ever-curious mind with a simple and effective strategy. The key, of course, is to make a habit of the strategy, and then it will continue to work.

Stoems - Hypno-learning

Hypno-learning is a way of integrating the information that you will be reading. The text that you will read in the hypno-learning passages following each section- I call them Stoems - will read like poetry. The design of the Stoems however has another and more potent design, that is to relax your mind and to help you to integrate the information that you have just read at a subconscious level. The passages will read something like:

So as I continue to read these words

continue to flow across

and

down

the page

as I relax

a little more

with each relaxing word

that's right

and noticing

as I blink

that's right

that I can read and learn

and continue to make

unconscious adjustments

so that I can feel relaxed

and calm

calm and relaxed

so I can continue to read

and wonder

and learn

effortlessly now.

that's right...

Did you blink? Most people notice that they blink and feel a little more relaxed as they read the words. This is because the passage you just read is 'pacing'[2] your experience of reading, and by doing so, it is inviting your conscious mind to be more in tune with your subconscious mind.

Blinking for example, is a subconscious process. By bringing your awareness to that process while you read, we are effectively suggesting that you relax a little deeper into that subconscious state of awareness.

Read the Stoems slowly and free of judgement or expectation, that way the words you read can and will lull you into a relaxed, open and receptive state of mind so you can continue learning easily now.

---

[2] *Talking about the thing that you are doing, i.e. reading*

Chapter 1

Wonder

> I have often wondered
>
> about my mind and body
>
> are connected
>
> in such an intimate and
>
> profound way
>
> I can continue to notice
>
> that as I read each relaxing word
>
> > That's right...
>
> I may continue to notice
>
> this wondering
>
> > and wandering
>
> with each confident word
>
> I can continue to relax
>
> and consider how well I can learn
>
> to just let go
>
> more and more
>
> deeply

and even

deeper...

stillness

comfortably reading

and wondering

as I let go

and continue to effortlessly

learn.

Chapter 2

The Problem with 'Sleep'

The distinctions we make between who we are and what we do can make the difference between being able to make changes in our lives, or not.

Let's get the ball rolling with a few questions.

1. Are you an insomniac or are you simply having difficulty sleeping?

2. Is there something wrong with you, or are you having difficulty sleeping?

The reason I am asking you these questions is simple; I would like you to consider that this thing called the 'sleeping problem' or 'insomnia' is something that you are doing, it has nothing to do with who you are. It's a behaviour that requires re-balancing, rather than being a fault in you.

Who you are is not what you do, think, or feel because what you do, think, or feel are 'behaviors' that are constantly changing over time. Who you are, the essential you, never changes, not at the deepest levels.

I would like you to consider that this sleeping challenge is something that you have been doing – and I guess you have been doing it very well – or you would not be reading this book.

To add to that, you would not be reading this book if you believed that someone else was going to fix this problem for you, which means of course, that you are in the process of fixing this sleeping challenge right now, as you read. That's right. And because you are continuing to read, you are continuing to understand that only you can fix this problem for yourself because it is you that has been 'doing' the problem.

We are the one 'doing' the problem, and it is up to us to undo, heal or resolve that problem.

There are many persuasive forces in life that can influence us and our thinking, feelings and our physical health, and yet regardless of what happens out there in the world around us, it is our interpretation of those events that turn them into something that is meaningful to us. Sleep is no different. Sleep is something that we do naturally and it is influenced by the comings and goings of life and how we respond to them.

It can be a relief to know that the challenge you have been having with sleep is nothing to do with who you are, it is simply a behaviour, an unconscious program (habit) that is changeable. And because you are the one who has been doing the sleep problem, then who could be better equipped to fix it now than you?

So as you continue to read and maybe even adjust your curiosity up a notch or two..., that's right, I would like you to make a picture in your mind.

Picture yourself 15 minutes after waking up from a fabulous deep sleep.

That's it.

Make this picture warm, joyful and empowering.

Take this picture and make a snap shot of it in your mind - about 10 x 8 inches, in full colour and hang it on a peg in the back of your mind. Later on I will explain in detail why this is so important.

Chapter 2

Distinctions

As I am reading

these comforting words

   that's right...

I can continue to consider...

that the problem I have been having

is just a behaviour

which means of course

that as I continue to read effortlessly now

   that's right...

I can take a deep breath...

and as I breathe out now...

   that's it...

I can continue to consider

that I am much more

than this problem ever was

just an old behaviour

that is already beginning to dissolve

                    into the past

                    behind me now

                    because, as I read on

                    comfortably

                            and easily

                                    that's it

            I am also moving forward

                            with ease

            and realising my ability to create

            a new way of thinking

            that continues to inspire me

            and surprise me

                    in many new ways

            I know that I am in the process now

            of leaving the old problem

                    is now behind me…

            and more and more

Chapter 2 — Better Sleep Sooner

I can continue to relax...

and enjoy learning

about my mind

and I don't

Mind...

Chapter 3

The Fascination Principle

Stories from childhood can be so inspirational. A friend told me a story that had a hidden meaning.

"When I was a boy," he began, "I would visit my Grandparent's house on the weekends. As I walked into their house and down the hall I would pass a tall and austere Grandfather Clock. From the moment I first encountered this monument to time I was spellbound."

"I would stand in front of its huge noisy presence and marvel at its mysterious nature, its endless chant, its persistent devotion to the invisible God - time."

"On one of these days, my Grandfather approached me carrying a chair which he promptly stood beside the Grandfather Clock. He then proceeded to move the clock out from the wall and to place the chair behind it. With a

twinkle in his eye he invited me to stand on the chair as he began to open up the back of the clock. The back of the clock swung open and inside was a circus of spinning and twisting, gleaming and turning, such a sight as I had never seen before. I was fascinated."

"*Every movement seemed somehow connected to every other movement and yet each individual part had a size and a shape and what appeared to be a singular purpose of its own. Every part working to a complex rhythm of its own and of the whole.*"

"*My Grandfather at once said, 'See that spring in there? It is wound so tight and it keeps the wheels turning, each wheel tight against the next. You can't change the movement of the clock by touching any of those big wheels or cogs or by trying to play with the spring, the tension is too great.'*"

"*Then all of a sudden he poked his finger through a gap in the turning circus of wheels and gently touched a spinning wheel that seemed to be made out of the lightest, finest gold, and all of a sudden, the clock slowed down and, for a moment, stopped.*"

"*I was holding my breath when my Grandfather said, "Even the most complex mechanism can be changed with the smallest touch.""*

I did not know until many years later that my friend's Grandfather was talking about the 'Butterfly Effect' or what is known in chaos theory as 'Sensitive Dependence'. Sensitive Dependence states that a small change at any one place in a complex system can have large effects somewhere else in the system and eventually can change the way the entire system operates.

I often wonder if the influence of a curious state of mind is very much like the gentle touch that my friend's Grandfather applied to the spinning wheel. Our curious attitude can immediately change the way we perceive an experience, and so, in our mind the experience has been transformed. And if the experience has changed in our mind, then the experience has changed for us.

Asthma as Teacher

Curiosity is the hand of Love that tickles our lives into animation.

The strangest awarenesses can occur during the most mundane tasks. I remember hearing that Einstein would often set a question to his subconscious and then go about doing something mundane and unrelated, later to be awakened form the trance of the mundane activity by the answer to that question.

While mowing the lawn one Spring morning, I developed a strategy that enabled me to release the frustrating illness known as asthma. It was a complete surprise to me at the time, considering I was an expert in asthma and had been since I was 4 years old. What I discovered through the release process was a strategy that could be applied to so many areas in life. I called this strategy *The Fascination Principle*, the title of my first book.

In a nutshell, *The Fascination Principle* is a three step process which swiftly moves a person from an unresourceful position of fear or worry to a state of healing. The strategy easily engages the ever-curious mind and redirects its immense creative power effortlessly inward so that it may find the resources to heal.

I incorporate *The Fascination Principle* in all areas of my work and when it comes to sleep, The Fascination Principle is a powerful ally. When we choose to engage the challenge of poor sleep or insomnia with a state of curiosity, the mind immediately opens up to deep internal wisdom, resources and possible outcomes that would normally have been invisible to us due to fear or worry.

The Fascination Principle considers all symptoms as a sign that healing is in motion. The symptom can be described as the subconscious mind communicating intelligently with our conscious mind, continuously giving us feedback and often asking for new suggestions.

The symptom, no matter what it is, may now be seen as a healthy and wise messenger that we can interact with in order to be inspired towards healing. All that is required is an attitude of curiosity.

Insomnia and poor sleep are symptoms of a behavioural imbalance at some level within us. This imbalance is being presented as sleeplessness, a symptom that when acknowledged with an open and curious attitude, can be redirected towards healing, not only of the symptoms, also the deeper imbalance.

The *Better Sleep Sooner* strategies that you will discover within this book have been designed primarily by looking at the symptoms of sleeplessness as symptoms of healing, and so, opportunities to heal. By employing *The Fascination Principle* we have been able to generate and identify new ways of looking at – 'reframing' – the symptoms of sleeplessness and directing those symptoms towards healing, and ...a *Better Sleep Sooner*.

Reframing Symptoms

    And a strategy

    for a better sleep

    inspires me to continue reading

    easily and confidently now

    I can just allow myself to consider

    with each relaxing word

    and each passing breath…

        that's right…

    that symptoms are a sign

    from deep

        down

            within me

    that I am continuing to balance

        and

            rebalance

    with ease

Chapter 3   **Better Sleep Sooner**

    my subconscious mind

    is continuously

    and effortlessly communicating

    as I continue to listen

    more and more easily now

    as I read

    and continue to wonder

    how I can easily notice

    that as I continue to read on

    effortlessly now

    I can continue to connect

    with my deeper wisdom

    continues to influence my ability to learn

    and to notice

        more and more

    how naturally sleep

    returns to my life

        as I relax a little deeper

and recognise that my body knows

more than I think it knows

as I feel it relaxing

ever deeper

and ever more purposefully

as I read on

and continue to learn more

                      that's right...

Chapter 4

The Power of Emotions

So often we fear the unseen and we imagine all manner of possible ongoing issues when in fact the way we respond to the symptoms of healing or any change for that matter will always set the stage for the process that follows.

Because I have been working with clients experiencing sleep problems for many years, I have noticed that emotions have a powerful influence on our ability to sleep. Emotions drive us. They are fuel for our minds and bodies and can be motivating one moment and demotivating the next. The emotions we feel generally rely upon our thoughts and beliefs for their fuel.

I find it so fascinating that we can feel such powerful emotions about thoughts or ideas that exist only in our minds. Our bodies do not know the difference between reality or fantasy and that is how we can remember a beautiful memory and feel a strong happy emotion. The opposite is also true.

There is a self-perpetuating circular process where emotions create sleeplessness and sleeplessness creates emotions and so on. Sleeplessness can generate very strong emotional responses such as anger and disappointment, and these emotions can in effect fuel the sleeping issue.

Anxiety is an emotion that can have very negative influences on our sleep, and of course, anxiety is one emotion that so many people experience when they have had a deficit of sleep. Anxiety is a fear of something happening – or not happening - in the future, and in this case, sleep. Anxiety is where we imagine the worst-case future scenarios and imagine it as if we are right there. This anxiety may come from lack of sleep in the past, which in turn begins to keep us awake at night, which in turn becomes fuel for more anxiety.

When we are able to acknowledge and resolve the emotions that are circulating within us and fueling the sleeplessness, we can return to a more balanced state of mind and body, and our sleep can return to what is normal for us.

A Powerful Key to Emotional Healing

Many years back, while investigating and discovering the cause of my body's illness and the healing that followed I became aware of a phenomenon that has continued to give my clients and myself a head start on the healing process.

To put it simply:

The emotion you are feeling about the challenge that you are facing, may be the emotion that is fueling that challenge.

Research in the field of psycho-neuro-immunology suggests that the emotions we feel will influence our body in the place where that emotion lives. In Chinese medicine for example, anger or frustration relates to the liver and that may be where the phrase "he was 'livid' (livered) at me" comes from.

Now, if the liver is out of balance it will generally give physical symptoms of that imbalance. Following that we will often begin to 'feel' something about the symptoms, often anger or frustration for example. In turn these emotions can perpetuate or create an imbalance in the liver.

What emotions do you experience when you cannot sleep? How do you feel about this challenge that you are having with sleep?

When you are able to acknowledge and identify the emotions that you are feeling about sleeplessness, then it is generally possible to release that emotion and then positively influence your ability to sleep.

There are many tools one can use for emotional release. Following are techniques that many of my clients have found invaluable when releasing the 'charge' of negative emotions.

Emotional Release Techniques

The Fascination Principle

Changing your mental state or perception with respect to your emotions is an important first step in resolving any emotion that may be fueling the sleeping problem.

The shift from a narrow or destructive mental state such as frustration or anger to an open, creative and expansive mental state, can be the difference between ongoing pain and surprising resolution and happiness.

So often, the answer that we seek is discovered in the most unlikely moments. As I mentioned in Chapter 2, I *was* an expert in creating asthma attacks. The weather, sometimes, stress, sometimes pollen in the air, or simply realising that I did not have my inhaler with me was all that was required to trigger my internal asthma mechanism into action. I was an expert in the art of asthma, and I hated it.

It was one day, a few months after completing my Clinical Hypnosis training, in the baking hot, Summer sun and while mowing the lawn, that I cured myself of asthma. completely! This is what happened:

As I said, I was mowing the lawn when the asthmatic symptoms began. This would normally signal the beginning of a slippery slope into an hour or two of discomfort, and yet, in that moment instead of traveling down the well worn track of frustration, fear and anxiety - emotions that fuel asthma - I noticed that I was appreciating this experience with curiosity. I was truly fascinated for the first time by this process of asthma. This, as you can imagine, was a major breakthrough.

Following that, I also realised that regardless of the apparent causes and influencing factors, (heat, pollen, exercise, etc) all of which could be contributing to the asthma, I was the only one *creating* the symptoms. I was '*doing*' them, and even though I was doing them subconsciously, I recognised that this 'doing' must be using strategies and processes to manifest the asthma - and to do it very well!

This realisation was followed by the awareness that my mind/body system is infinitely intelligent - a network of intelligence designed to learn, heal and grow, - and that it was generating these symptoms as a response to the healing process. I recalled times when I had cut or grazed myself and there was always a 'symptom' of the healing process such as bleeding, which was generally followed by the forming of a scab and then a light scar. I did not question this process, it was a natural part of my life.

This being the case it also occurred to me that the way we learn how to respond to the healing process is primarily through suggestions. Suggestions from people around us and of course from the suggestions we make to ourselves, and the only suggestions I had ever offered my subconscious mind about asthma were based on fear and drama.

So, for the first time in my life I made a decision about what I wanted, not what history would dictate. With that I began to wonder;

"I wonder how I am continuing to heal myself now so I can finish the lawn and then go to the beach with the dogs - feeling happy."

At that point I imagined throwing a stick for my two dogs on the beach.

45 minutes later, while bending down to switch off the mower, I realised that I had not had the asthma. I had dissolved the asthma attack and I felt as light as a feather. The end of asthma!

There are three key points to *The Fascination Principle* Strategy:

1. Acknowledge the emotion/symptom: "I feel [angry] because I cannot sleep".

2. Generate a state of curiosity: "This is fascinating" or simply; "Wow!"

3. Initiate the internal healing process: "I wonder how, I am continuing to resolve this [anger] now, so that I can relax and rest deeply so I can wake up feeling refreshed in the morning."

Fundamentally, I believe that our minds are in a constant state of insatiable curiosity. Curiosity is a powerful state of mind which effortlessly empowers and motivates us, giving us a compelling nudge the right direction in order to generate change and wellbeing.

Remember, all of our learning is stimulated by the constant stream of suggestions from external sources. The suggestions we make to ourselves, the thoughts and feelings we have about those experiences became our learnings. All we need to do is take control of the suggestions we make to ourselves in order to generate change, happiness and well being.

You can get a deeper understanding of *The Fascination Principle* by reading my book '*Rapid Inspired Change, Turn Symptoms into Well being using The Fascination Principle*'.

Emotional Freedom Technique

Emotional Freedom Technique (EFT) is a simple and effective strategy for dissolving negative emotions. It works on the emotional energy pathways of the body (meridians) to release emotions easily and quickly by tapping specific pressure points on your own body.

Refer to the appendix for EFT instructions.

Self Hypnosis

The ability to relax at will is an essential tool that enables the mind and body to re-balance and release old unwanted stress and emotions. Self-Hypnosis is primarily a relaxation tool using specific techniques to bypass the 'chatter' of the mind and to help the mind and body to relax and rejuvenate. Adding positive statements and emotions to this relaxation process gives Self-Hypnosis its power.

SelfhHypnosis is so effective because when we are enjoying a deeply relaxed state of mind we are more able to receive and integrate new ideas. The subconscious mind, during deep relaxation, is more open to compelling suggestions and when these suggestions are aligned with our highest intentions and repeated over time, they become part of our internal programming.

Self-Hypnosis in its most simple application is a powerful way to relax. What could be better.

Refer to the appendix for a Self-Hypnosis script and instructions.

Rewind the Day

Rewind the Day is a fantastic tool for slowing down the mind and releasing any tension that may be hanging over from the day. Children love it as well.

We effortlessly accept the idea of emotions moving 'forward' in time because emotions are connected to events. When we run events backwards however, it is difficult to feel the emotions of those events, and with that we lose the attachments to those events. Emotions and the attachment to those emotions work in forward motion, not in reverse.

Imagine a horror movie being rewound and all of the events occur in reverse. The entire movie becomes comical and weird rather than frightening.

Interestingly this rewinding process has successfully been incorporated into an NLP strategy named the Trauma/Phobia cure.

So, when lying in bed at night, or just before you get into bed, imagine the day in reverse. Run it backwards. Imagine it 'through your own eyes' from the last thing you did backwards through the day to the first thing you did after getting out of bed that morning.

Try to see as much detail as you can. Every now and then you will notice that you have missed bits out, that is ok, keep going backwards to the start. Then do it again. Run the process two or three times if you can. Running your day in reverse can often cause you to drift into sleep... which is a nice surprise.

For children Reversing the Day is a wonderful way to release any 'sticky' emotions, or locked up energy from the day. It is a bit like a 'de-brief' for the ever curious mind. The way that consistently works for children is to do it with them while they are lying in bed.

For example:

"Before we got into bed, we brushed our teeth…"

"before we brushed our teeth we…"

Reversing the Day is such a simple strategy and as I alluded to earlier this process of rewinding the day can also be used to rewind an event.

Some events can stick like glue. After an unexpected event we can continue to feel emotionally affected and attached to that event long after it is over. A powerful way to release the emotional attachment is to rewind it three or four times.

Start at the point just after the event has finished and rewind it to the point just before the event began. Repeat this process until you can feel that something is different about the way you think and feel about the event. Rewinding the event while whistling carousel or circus music can add a 'unique' edge to the process which will definitely change the way it feels. You will be amazed at how it works.

Curious State

        I have been reading about curiosity

        and how I can turn curiosity

        into wellbeing

        and that means

        I can continue to consider

        with every inspired word

        that there have been times in my life

        where I have been inspired

        to change my mind

        and create new ideas

              rise effortlessly

                    like bubbles of curiosity

        that I am now connecting with

        my inner creativity and curiosity

        more and more easily now

        I can notice the feelings of inspiration

Chapter 4 — Better Sleep Sooner

as I read and wonder

how I am continuing

to turn this information

into useful and powerful tools

that I can keep on using

when I am in bed

it is curious to consider

and yet some how obvious

that at the deepest levels

    of my mind

is in a constant state of curiosity...

and as I continue to read

and drift a little more

    that's right

into this curious

    and dreamy state

of relaxation and wonder

how quickly I am integrating

all that I need

right now

so I can easily allow

the natural process of sleep

to become a welcome

and effortless part of my life

now.

Chapter 5

Reframing the Sleep Process

The key to the *Better Sleep Sooner* strategies is reframing. Reframing is where we take a look at a challenge, issue or idea from more than the one and often familiar point of view. We see the challenge through a different frame. Similar to viewing a painting, the frame in which the painting is presented can change the perception we have of the painting.

Seeing the symptom as the beginning of the healing process rather than the beginning of an illness, for example, is a reframe. This reframe gives us an opportunity to expand our choices, giving us more openness with respect to how we experience our lives.

Changing the frame through which we view the sleep process can have a profound influence on our ability to drift off into a deep and restful sleep. Suddenly the experiences that we were feeling challenged about become doorways that lead us to where we want to be. When we reframe our experiences we simply have more choices available to us.

The importance of Rest

Rest is so important and as I will discuss later in this chapter, rest could be one of the most important reframes you could possible make with regards to getting to sleep easily at night. However in this instance the rest I am talking about is the rest that you take during the day. The rest that you will take during the day will have a profound influence on your sleeping experience at night.

Having practiced meditation and self-hypnosis for the last 20 years, I have experienced the unquestionable influence that these practices can have on life and sleep. Meditation and self-hypnosis both take the mind to a more 'coherent' state; a state of relaxation and calm. When the mind enters such a state of coherence and calm, the body naturally follows. The deeper we take our mind into relaxation the deeper is the relaxation and calm experienced by the body. The body simply follows the instructions of the mind.

When the mind and body relax deeply, tension is released, and as tension releases the mind and body naturally release stored stress. Releasing stored stress as we relax is a natural process and is often the reason why we feel agitated when we start to relax in bed at night. I will discuss this challenge in greater detail later.

The healing and rejuvenating benefits of a short rest and relaxation period during the day are profound when creating a healthy lifestyle and excellent sleeping habits.

Taking the time each day to meditate or practice self-hypnosis creates the mental and physical space to release stress easily. By taking this time we are effectively reducing the amount of stress that we take to bed with us at night, therefore reducing the amount of 'de-stressing' we experience as we relax in bed.

Power-napping, nano or 'nana' napping are other terms used to describe day time rest. Taking short power-naps can have an immediate result; more energy, clarity and patience to name a few. The difference between a 'nap' and meditation or Self-Hypnosis is that more often than not we tend to fall asleep in a nap. This is beneficial as long as the naps are short and not too close to bed time. The same can be said for meditation or Self-

Hypnosis. Practiced too close to bed time and the energising or stimulating effects of the practice may cause sleeplessness.

There is no 'one' solution with regards to meditation or Self-Hypnosis, it is a personal choice. What I have noticed in my own experience is that a combination of meditation and Self-Hypnosis is beneficial. Finding a form of meditation that works for you may take a little investigation and *will* require some commitment.

Self-Hypnosis is easy to learn, requires only the amount of time that you are willing to devote to it each day and is focussed on the outcome you want, for example, feeling more energised. Self-Hypnosis is not generally considered a spiritual practice and seldom discussed in the same breath as enlightenment and higher states of consciousness and yet by its very nature – inducing a trance state – Self-Hypnosis is indeed a very spiritual and enlightening practice. As stated earlier, the only real difference between Hypnosis and Meditation is that hypnosis tends to be more focused on a specific outcome. If you want hypnosis to be more spiritual then that is the focus you need to have when practicing it.

Interestingly, even though Meditation is a little less focused with respect to the outcome it can be very focussed in its practice. Practicing Meditation generally requires a commitment of at least 20 minutes twice a day to get the full benefit. Meditation can be very uplifting, relaxing, healing, enlightening and yet it can also be hard work, repetitious and demanding, that said, in my experience, worth every moment devoted to it.

Above all, the practice of taking rest during the day is very beneficial and regardless of what strategy or strategies you choose, you are guaranteed that your life will become more calm and your sleep... well, you will wake up each morning feeling refreshed.

Refer to the appendix for a Self-Hypnosis script and also a description of how to run a short and sweet 'power-nap'.

Reframe 1 - Did I Sleep?

Bed is prepared. Atmosphere created. Attitude of expectation. Sleep is invited, never enforced.

So many clients lament their lack of sleep. Like a long lost friend, sleep has abandoned them and is no longer a reliable and welcome visitor. If this sounds familiar, then I want you to answer these questions: has sleep not visited lately, or have you only recognised the being awake moments and generalised those to meaning - "I didn't get any sleep?"

Generalising lack of sleep is easy to do because all we can be aware of during the night is the times when we are awake, everything else is sleep, which of course is unconscious.

Why is this important? It so happens that the beliefs we have about sleep have a huge influence on our ability to sleep and the effectiveness of the sleep that we do get.

There is no definitive science to decipher the mystery about how much sleep is the right amount. Many times I have had a few hours sleep and felt great the next day. On the other hand I have also had 10 hours sleep and felt less than fabulous the next day.

I want you to consider that there could be many possible variations on the amount of sleep that you need from day to day and your requirements will change from day to day depending on many variables such as food, stress, general health and more.

Also consider that the times you wake up are the only times that you are 'conscious' during the night, and just because you're awake does not mean that you are not getting enough sleep. In fact all it means is that you are awake at that moment. That's it.

Consider that the times when you are awake in the night are times when your body/mind system have awoken for a reason, such as to get more comfortable, or a dream was very active, or there has been a lot on your mind, or there is stress in your nervous system or you just need to pee.

The more you allow yourself to reframe the conscious moments in the night as nothing more than what they are - conscious moments, and to allow your inner wisdom to define how much sleep you need, the sooner you will be able to make the most of the time you spend in bed. The truth is, you have possibly been sleeping <u>more</u> than not during the night...

    and this means

    that I can continue to consider more

    and more

    as I continue to read

    more

Chapter 5 — Better Sleep Sooner

and relax

a little deeper now

that I have often slept

when I may have thought

that I had not

and yet I can continue to recognise

with each passing breath

    that's right

that I have slept

    and rested

deeply enough to know

that I know how to relax

    and rest

        deeply

more and more

confidently just letting go

as I continue to learn

that sleep

is a natural experience

that I can continue to remember

to let go

with confidence and ease

and let it happen

      more effortlessly

now...

Reframe 2 - Rest or Sleep?

Lisa's Story

Lisa came to a workshop I was presenting. Lisa sleeps very well and yet the entire time she is listening and making notes, she is aware of her husband and his sleeplessness.

Working as a hypnotherapist, she had wondered many times how she could help her husband sleep and yet she did not know where to start.

A few weeks after the worksop I received an email from Lisa and it read;

"Hi Aaron. When I returned home from the long day of the workshop and I could remember straight away that sleep is not the problem and that rest is the key. So I told my husband what I thought you had said and you know what? For the first time in months he fell asleep and slept through the night."

~//~

One of the most important reframes occurred on the night I had 'The Sleep Epiphany' some 20 years ago.

I was lying in bed driving myself to literal distraction with worry and thoughts and most destructively, a continuous internal dialogue that went something like:

"WHY AM I NOT ASLEEP?... WHY CAN I NOT GO TO SLEEP?... WHEN WILL I GO TO SLEEP?... and AHHHHHHH I AM GOING INSANE!"

Know the feeling?

Then all of a sudden, a miracle happened. In the middle of the mental madness and monkey mind chatter I asked myself the weirdest question: "How will I know if I am asleep?" to which I immediately answered: "I won't!"

And then I noticed that my left knee... stay with me here... I realised that my left knee was 'resting', yes, you read it right, my left knee was resting. At that instant I also realised that many other parts of my body were in a state of increasing rest or restfulness. In that moment I generated a little self-dialogue about my experience along the lines of; "I am resting... my knee is resting... my arms are resting..." and so on.

The next thing I knew, I was waking up to the sound of the ocean, and birdsong, and with the first real feeling of energy that I had had in months. I was amazed because it was the following morning.

The most powerful and effective reframe that you can create right now is to <u>change sleep</u> – an experience you will never 'consciously' have – <u>into rest</u> – an experience that you do consciously experience - with an element of ease.

Sleep is a conscious unknown because we are not consciously aware of it. Sleep is an event that we know we will drift into at some point, and following that, at some unknown time we will effortlessly wake up from it. Rest, however, is an experience that we can 'calibrate'. We can notice it and be aware of how much, or how little of it we are having. Rest is conscious to us and that means we can continue to notice it until its delicious invitation brings sleep.

Chapter 5 — Better Sleep Sooner

Resting is an experience that we can consciously enjoy. Rest is an experience that has no stress attached to it and has a profound and healthy influence on our mind and body. So...

    as I continue to read comfortably

    and calmly now

    I can begin to reframe sleep

    into resting and

        relaxing

            deeper

    as I continue to notice

    that parts of my body feel rested

        and relaxed

            right now

    that's right

    I can notice that I feel relieved

    to consider

    that when I lie in bed

    I can continue to relax and rest

ever so deeply

and with every effortless breath

    that's right...

I continue to allow my mind

    and body

with each and every gentle word

to make some subtle adjustments

deep down inside now

    that's right

so that when I imagine being in bed

I notice I feel more and more accepting

    and grateful

for this amazing process of resting

    deeper and

        deeper

that's it...

knowing that at some point

I will awaken effortlessly

relaxed and refreshed...

Reframe 3 - The internal sleep conflict.

Following on from 'Reframe 2' - "when was the last time you had a conscious experience of sleep?"

As previously stated, it is not normally possible to experience sleep consciously because sleep is unconscious. Because sleep is unconscious it does not make any sense to lie in bed wondering why you are not asleep or wondering when you will get to sleep, because you will never know. By lying in bed fretting over the sleep dilemma we are effectively creating a conflict between the conscious and the unconscious. We are trying to speak the language of sleep without the knowledge of that language.

The idea that sleep is something that you don't have to think about anymore is a major breakthrough. I realised this myself one night when I was about to say to my daughter; "Just roll over and go to sleep". I caught myself in time and rephrased the comment immediately to a statement that she could understand and do, and that was; "Roll over darling, close your eyes and rest and while you're resting picture yourself tomorrow, just after waking up, feeling happy." We can create the environment that invites sleep, and yet we cannot 'make' sleep happen.

Thinking about the 'how' and 'when' of sleep creates an inner conflict between your conscious desire and your unconscious process because at a conscious level we are trying to do something that we do not <u>do</u> consciously and this can perpetuate a belief that we can't sleep…

> and that means
>
> that as I continue
>
> to enjoy reading to myself now
>
> > that's right
>
> comfortably and confidently
>
> I can imagine resting in my bed now
>
> > that's it
>
> and as I continue to read and imagine
>
> I can notice that I am not asleep yet
>
> and that is OK now
>
> as I continue to notice
>
> that I am aware

that at some point

    I will drift and doze

into sleep

    that's right

and then after that

at some point

I will wake up refreshed

and this means

    that I can continue to relax

and learn comfortably

as I notice that I am reading

    and resting...

    that's right...

I am resting,

and this is relaxing

    and comforting

to know that I can just let go

    and relax and rest

as new learnings and understandings

continue to preserve themselves

deep inside

I can continue to feel

more and more rested

as I realise that sleep

is no longer an issue

as I notice that I can feel relaxed

about resting deeper

and effortlessly content

now

Reframe 4 - Sleep - Path or Destination?

Sleep is not a destination!

When I ask clients with sleep issues what they want, obviously they reply that they want to sleep. Although this is a fair enough answer, it is not an answer that is useful to them, simply because sleep is not a destination.

A destination is place that we can appreciate and experience with our senses when we reach it, and as we have already discussed, because sleep is unconscious we will not know when we have reached it.

Sleep is a process and a pathway to something else. The destination or the outcome that we are really looking for is not sleep. The destination is what we notice after sleep, it is the next day, after we wake up. The destination of course is the next day, feeling alert, rested and happy.

So, when you think of sleep, think of it as an unconscious journey. The process of sleep is like a drive to the shop to buy a few groceries. On the way to the shop you are operating the car automatically and mostly from unconscious habit. Once you return home, you cannot remember very much about the processes that were involved in the driving experience. Your purpose was to get home with the groceries, and everything else was taken care of by your faithful and reliable subconscious mind.

So the destination or 'outcome' you are after is the feeling that occurs after a good night's sleep. The feeling of rejuvenation, feeling relaxed, clear headed, motivated and so on.

Remember back to the beginning of this book and the image I asked you to create in your mind. The image of yourself, 15 minutes after waking up from a blissful sleep. Take that image again now and make it bright, colourful and inviting. Make it so 'yummy' that you just want to have it now. This is your destination and you will know what it is like when you get there. So…

    I don't mind considering

    for a few relaxing moments

    that I know more

        than I think I know

    how to let go and relax

        more and more

    as I read and wonder

        that's right

    just how easily I can continue to read

        and learn

            and relax deeper

    and notice that every comfortable word

    reminds me that

Chapter 5 — Better Sleep Sooner

I do not mind

remembering that sleep is a process

that I can consciously forget

    that's right

as I continue to remember now

that the reason for lying in bed

    and resting

so that I can wake up every morning

    feeling refreshed

        that's right...

as I restfully read on

    that's right

and notice

that with every breath

    that's it

I can continue to consider

    the deeper ways

I am changing the way I think

about sleep

happens automatically

like blinking now

    that's right

I know I can relax deeper

    and really notice

that the idea of inviting sleep

    is already feeling easier

    ahhhh…

    what a relief.

Chapter 5

Reframe 5 - The 'Healing Feelings'.

Mark's Story

Sometimes, when met with an almost insurmountable challenge, the subconscious mind reveals yet another layer of genius.

As a young boy Mark endured a significant degree of abuse. It started at the age of 4 years old and continued for many years. It did not matter what he did to try to 'do the right thing', any attempt at connection was met with anger.

One night after a 'beating' Mark was lying in bed in agony and in tears. He had a movie playing over and over in his mind, tirelessly repeating the events of the day. It was as if he was watching a re-run over and over and with every repetition he subsided deeper and deeper into despair.

Suddenly, out of nowhere, like in a dream, a TV set materialised and hovered in front of him, just within arms reach. On the TV screen the memories of the day were playing. The movie that had been playing in his mind was repeating when suddenly, and to the right of the screen, like on any TV set, he noticed the channel switch. Mark reached up grabbed hold of the channel switch and changed channel. That night and from that night onwards the pain subsided and sleep's warm embrace encased him till morning. Finally Mark had a strategy for safety and the opportunity to rest.

~//~

Mark's story is extraordinary and yet it tells us something very important; we can heal and we can surprise ourselves in the ways that we do it.

As we begin to relax in bed, we also begin a very important and yet often unrecognised and misunderstood processes; the processes of releasing stress and tension, the processes of healing and rejuvenation.

The challenge that so many of us have when lying in bed is what to do with the symptoms of these resting processes.

One of the most effective ways of releasing the tension and frustration that these symptoms bring is to change the way we think about them.

In some yogic traditions, there is an understanding that comes with regular meditation, and that is, "sensations are just sensations". We notice them, we are aware of them and yet we give them little energy and certainly no judgement or emotion. We simply acknowledge them as a Release of Stress, a symptom of the body rebalancing.

My experience with meditation has shown me and many meditators that more often than not sensations such as twitches and itching are the "dark forces" that disrupt our rest and have the potential to stop us from relaxing and journeying within. These 'road blocks' to inner awareness exist however, not because of the sensations we are experiencing, but because of our responses to those sensations.

Uncomfortable feelings or unusual sensations can become maddening if we don't know what they really mean and what to do with them. In a nutshell, sensations are a sign that we are continuing to relax and heal, and as we continue to relax and heal, the accumulated stress, energy or emotional tension that has been sitting within us begins to release.

We now know that sensations are an important and valuable part of our resting process. Almost like a right-of-passage to greater awareness in meditation, sensations that occur while we are in bed resting can be respectfully viewed as a significant and important sign that we are relaxing, healing and moving ever deeper into the unconscious bliss of sleep. Which means…

as I continue to read comfortably

      and easily

considering the new learnings

and understandings

about sensations

as I let go

      more and more

I can comfortably allow myself to relax

      even deeper now

and wonder…

      that's right

really wonder

how I am continuing to reframe

my moment to moment experiences

are constantly changing

      and reminding me

that I do not mind

simply letting go

    more and more easily

as I read

and imagine lying in bed

just noticing sensations

and how wonderful it is

to know

that I now know

    that I can relax deeper

with every comforting sensation

into a blissful acceptance

that nothing bothers me now

that I understand that sensations

are simply sensations

    come and go

        as I read and breathe

and blink

    that's right

I can continue to learn more

and it feels good

    to learn with ease

and confidently opening up to new

and fascinating ideas

help me to sleep like a baby

from this moment forward

I can look forward

    to rest

Reframe 6 - Thoughts, Bubbles in Champagne

    Wow, if there is one thing that can drive us crazy when we are lying in bed waiting to fall sleep, it is random or persistent thoughts and the accompanying internal dialogue. The droning repetition of thoughts and the constant internal responses:

Chapter 5 — Better Sleep Sooner

"I should be asleep!"

"Oh #%$ I am never going to be able to function tomorrow…"*

"Oh hell I have that meeting tomorrow…"

"Did I put the rubbish out?"

As I said earlier, sensations are a sign that your body is doing what it is designed to do when we begin the resting process. As soon as we begin to relax we are beginning to *release stress*.

The thoughts we experience while lying in bed awaiting sleep are no different in their nature to the sensations and twitches discussed earlier. The thoughts we notice are symptoms that our nervous system is successfully beginning to relax, heal, rejuvenate – and release stress.

Michael's Story

Michael worked in a very well respected IT company in Australia when the Global Financial Crisis (GFC) occurred. One day he was working in a secure and successful company and the next "the bottom fell out of everything".

Michael came to see me because he was not sleeping. He had taken initiative and turned the change in the market to his advantage by setting up a business which helped people in IT to tackle the problems faced by the ongoing GFC, and yet, even though his new business was doing well, he could not sleep.

"It's the thoughts. They are 10 to the dozen. Never stopping and so frustrating!"

Michael was reflecting on his personal experience, an experience that by no means is unique to him. Changing circumstances, insecurity and loss can have a huge influence on our ability to let go and relax. The stress that events such as the GFC can create is huge and often overwhelming. It can also mean that as soon as our head hits the pillow and we begin to relax, the unresolved challenges start to appear - and start screaming like screeching bats.

I asked Michael to think of the thoughts as a sign of the ongoing healing process that occurs when we begin to rest. Thoughts are a sign that healing is occurring and that the mind and body are 'sorting out' the junk of the day.

I asked Michael to close his eyes and to relax a little. I then asked Michael to remember lying in bed and to remember the last time he had those troubling thoughts, which was not difficult. I then asked him to remember the thoughts and to think of them as he would think of bubbles rising in champagne - just watch them rise, rest a moment and then disappear - just watch.

I offered a few more suggestions (that you will read about later) and I watched as Michael slumped into the chair and began to breathe very deeply.

Michael had two more sessions with me and has continued to drift into sleep easily every night. He reported recently that because he and his wife had moved house, he had had a few disruptions that historically would have disrupted his sleep, and yet, now that he knows what the thoughts mean, he simply drifts off to sleep regardless.

~//~

How many times have you noticed that the thoughts you have at night are about 'stuff' that was, or 'stuff' that might be, or completely random thoughts that have no apparent relevance? Well, these thoughts have a frequency or vibration that relates directly to the nature of the stress that is being released.

For example; as a stress related to an 'angry' event is released, the frequency of anger will influence the way the mind experiences that release of stress. What may follow is angry thoughts and possibly angry sensations.

Regardless of what nature the thoughts may take, the thoughts are a healthy sign of healing, balancing and rejuvenation. You are releasing stress and tension.

Think of the thoughts that come and go like bubbles rising from the bottom of a glass of champagne. We can see the bubbles materialise out of nowhere and then spontaneously rise to the surface, linger for a moment, and then POP! disappear. We don't go searching for the popped bubble, it is gone. We don't start wondering what that popped bubble was all about, or what kind of life it had or message it was trying to bring... it has popped and gone...

> and this is how
>
> we can continue to notice
>
> that's right
>
> that with every breath
>
> I can continue to wonder
>
> and wander

from word to effortless word

    sinking deeper

and more confidently now

into the depths

of my subconscious mind

knows exactly how

    to reframe thoughts

simply come and go

as effortlessly

    as I continue to notice

that I am breathing effortlessly

    that's it

and learning that thoughts are energy

rising into my awareness

like bubbles in champagne

as I continue to read

and relax

and wonder how quickly

I am continuing to notice

that I feel more

    and more relaxed

about thoughts and sensations

when I imagine lying in bed

    resting and relaxing

    with ease...

just allowing sleep to come

in its own perfect

and beautiful

    way

        Ahhhhhh....

Reframe 7 - Noisy sounds

Because we originally lived a more 'primitive' life in the natural world where wild creatures, wild people and wild storms, dinosaurs, aliens, and other scary things could wreck havoc upon our lives, when we closed our eyes at night our other senses would intensify in order to make sure that we continued to be safe. Nothing has changed.

At night, while lying in bed and drifting off, our natural subconscious programming for self preservation kicks in and our ears intensify their acuity in order to keep us safe. This of course means that we are often much more aware of sounds inside and outside our bedroom at night.

Our greater sensitivity to sound at night is a sign that we are doing what we are designed to do… and that we are doing it very well.

When I was suffering from sleepless nights, I would invariably find myself thinking about all the noises that I could hear. I was living near a well populated beach which had many visitors day and night. Like many, I would lie in bed unable to shift my focus from the 'noises' I could not help hearing. Then one night, for no apparent reason

I decided that the noises were not noises at all. They were <u>sounds</u>.

You may have noticed that I have continued to use the word sound rather than the word noise. For argument's-sake, there is no noise – there is only sound. The two words, 'noise' and 'sound' describe an auditory event and yet there is a difference. The word 'noise' is sharp and even loud, while the word 'sound' is softer and somewhat comforting. The word noise seems uncontrollable while the word sound is malleable and forgiving, maybe even a little musical.

Melissa's Story

Melissa came to see me because she was not sleeping. She was feeling stressed and very upset. The reason she could not sleep was her husband's snoring. Melissa's husband snored from the moment he fell asleep until the moment he woke in the morning. She tried sleeping in another bed at the other end of the house and yet she could still hear the 'noise'.

I helped Melissa to relax and then I asked her to imagine being in bed resting and to notice that there were a few sounds outside the room, like crickets or the occasional passing car. I then asked her to notice that they were only sounds, coming and going. As she imagined this scenario, she began to relax even deeper.

I then asked her to imagine her husband getting into bed and to notice the sounds of her own breathing and to also notice that there was a sound that told her that her husband was soundly asleep and that it was simply a sound. That sound could simply become like all the other sounds that occur during the night - passing sounds that come and go as she relaxes deeper and deeper.

After a week, Melissa returned for a follow up session and told me that for the last two nights she had slept next to her husband and for some reason had not been bothered by the 'sound' of her husband snoring.

$$\sim//\sim$$

A sound becomes a noise because of what we believe about it and the meaning we give to it. It is always a sound and sounds come and go, weave and flow and we don't seem to mind.

Making this simple change can make a massive difference to our perception. We can take this new idea and begin to 'filter' our experience in an entirely new way - and that of course means...

it is natural to hear sounds

coming and going

effortlessly passing me by

as I read these confident words

    that's right

I notice sounds all about me now

    come and go

        passing by

like clouds in the sky

as I continue to read effortlessly

and relax softly

    softly relax

comfortably and confidently

noticing that I have reframed noise

into sounds

    flow effortlessly

day and night

I continue to feel more and more relaxed

and at ease

now that sounds

simply come and go

as I relax more and more

deeper and

        deeper

into complete calm

encompassing my thoughts

        and feelings

ever-changing experiences

that mean I can continue to consider

just how surprised I will be

when I wake up refreshed

        and rejuvenated…

Reframe 8 - The Falling Feeling

In seminars, one of the most frequent questions that I am asked is: "What is that falling feeling?"

You are lying in bed and you are beginning to relax and as you continue to relax, you can feel the sensations of letting go. You notice that you are drifting off... drifting... then ... all of a sudden you fall. It was like your entire body dropped a few feet into the bed. It does not matter how much you try to rationalise the experience, it felt like you were falling.

Similar to many other resting sensations or experiences, this 'falling' feeling is a sign that you are doing what you are designed to do when you begin to rest. The only difference this time is that you are doing it very fast.

Imagine for a moment that your conscious thoughts are like the waves rippling across the surface of the ocean. What lies beneath the waves are deeper and deeper levels of thought where the mind is more and more rested and quiet.

When we close our eyes we send a message to the brain to relax and slide into the deeper reaches of this ocean of consciousness. On occasion the slide from a conscious state into a deeper level of mental rest can be very fast. The body, being an extension of our thoughts, does not know the difference between reality and imagination, so when the mind slips deeply and often suddenly into the deeper reaches of rest and calm, the body 'feels' like it has fallen. The mental transition translates into a physical reality of falling.

To repeat; this is a positive sign that you are relaxing deeply and quickly and that you have released a chunk of tension that has allowed you to 'drop' into a deep rest. The challenge of course is that we are often woken or startled by the experience. The key here is to be curious and not mind at all... just continue to relax...

and as I continue to relax

and read

each effortless word

moves with ease

into my consciousness

knows the difference

between fantasy and reality

can feel different to my body

simply listens to my thoughts

come and go

with every gentle breath

      that's right

that comes and goes

I can continue to be aware

that every experience I notice

as I continue to rest

      and relax

relax and

rest

deeper now

I know that I can trust

that everything I need to know

to drift deeper into sleep

when the time is just right

I can relax and slip

      into a deep

and restful

    sleep.

Chapter 6

The Better Sleep Sooner Strategy

This strategy could not be easier and that is why I ask you to have an open mind and to remember that some of the most powerful and influential learnings that we have in our lives can come from a single and often innocent experience.

The strength of this strategy comes from a hypnotic process called *'Pace and Lead'*. This simply means that the strategy uses your moment-to-moment experience in order to create the restful experience that will lull you into sleep. Using the strategy you will be 'pacing' your moment-to-moment experiences in order to 'lead' yourself into the restful and sleepy state of mind.

This strategy is designed to be used whenever or wherever you need to rest and sleep. It is designed primarily as an 'internal dialogue' process and you will be talking to yourself about the experience of being in bed and by doing this you will be transforming the experience of being in bed into a state of restfulness that will help you to sleep.

Before we talk about the strategy, here are a few thoughts to consider that will make the strategy more effective.

Being 'In the Now'

A contributing factor of sleeplessness is that we are not present to the moment. We are always thinking about what has been and what may be. Worrying about the past or anxious about the future.

Being 'present' to the moment is essential when generating the experience of rest. When we are present to the moment, we are also present to our body and its natural inclination to rest.

The *Better Sleep Sooner* strategy ensures that you can continue to be present and aware of the moment-to-moment sensations and thoughts that will eventually lull you to sleep.

Releasing judgement - As it is

Being free of judgement can enable us to take each moment as it comes. When we are free of judgement the sensations of the body, the thoughts that rise or the sounds that appear can simply be what they are.

So many of our challenges in life arise because we continue to judge each experience rather than simply letting it be what it is. We challenge our moment-to-moment experience of life against our beliefs and this leads us away from the real fact that a thought is a thought, a sensation is a sensation and a sound is a sound.

While using the following strategy, leave judgement beside the bed for a while, pick it up later if you want it and yet while in bed resting, just let what happens, happen.

The only outcome you are considering as you lie in bed resting is the idea that you will be refreshed and revitalised when you awaken. Everything else is a transient visitor. Let it be as it is – we just don't mind.

Persist

No matter what you may initially think or feel about this strategy... keep going. I have had a few clients come to me and say... "I did what you said and I had to do it over and over and I just about went mad..."

Persist. The only reason it could be difficult to continue is simple: you will probably get caught up in your thought processes and judgements. Once you notice that you have been thinking, thinking, thinking, bla bla bla... just come back to the process.

Persistence and of course repetition are the parents of skill and so regardless of the thoughts or feelings, just notice them and then return to the strategy.

'And...'

You will notice that the word '_and_' is underlined throughout the strategy. This is the most important word in the strategy... believe it or not. It is important because it is 'inclusive'. Regardless of what your experience may be, by using '_and_' you are creating the link that will 'lead' that experience into deeper rest.

The Strategy

When lying in bed bring your awareness to the pillow and notice the sensation of the pillow against the side of your face or the back of your head. Notice the pillow, - and gently and warmly say to yourself:

"Ah... it feels so good to be in bed resting...

The pillow feels good...

<u>*and*</u> *here I am resting...*

It feels so good to be in bed resting..."

Now notice the sheets against your skin. The weight or lightness of the bedding, and say to yourself:

"The sheets feel good –

<u>*and*</u> *here I am resting..."*

Now notice a part of your body that is resting, e.g. your elbow:

"my elbow feels relaxed...

<u>*and*</u> *here I am resting..."*

Now notice your breathing. Notice the gentle inward breath and the gentle outward breath and simply be aware of your breath. Notice the sensation of the air passing through your nostrils as it comes in... and goes out. Think to yourself:

"Breathing gently …

gently breathing…"

At some point you may notice a sound, so say to yourself:

"There's a sound

<u>*and*</u> *here I am resting.*

It feels good to be resting."

You may notice a sensation in your body. You may notice a discomfort or itch. If it is something you can immediately resolve by itching or moving, do so and then say to yourself:

"There's a sensation – and here I am resting – the sheets feel good – the pillow feels relaxed – and I am resting."

Once again, be aware of your breathing…

"breathing gently

gently breathing…

<u>and</u> here I am… resting."

Sooner or later you will notice thoughts. You may even notice thoughts about this strategy – good – that means you are resting and relaxing and releasing stress. Say to yourself:

"There's a thought –

<u>and</u> here I am resting…

thoughts come and go

<u>and</u> I am resting."

It is so good to be in bed resting".

Keep this gentle and non-judgmental internal dialogue flowing.

Thoughts and doubts may appear so:

"There's a thought

    <u>and</u> here I am resting."

Come back to your breathing…You can think to your self,

"breathing gently -

    gently breathing…"

and continue…

Remain equanimous – calm and even-tempered. Simply do not mind the experiences <u>and</u> that means you can continue to notice…

    I am reading these words

    comfortably and easily

as they flow across

and

down

the page

and with ease

I can continue to consider

all that I have read

has already preserved itself

deep within

I can consider that as I read more

I can continue to notice

with every gentle breath

that's right

that I can imagine

lying in my bed

and relaxing deeper

Chapter 6 — Better Sleep Sooner

I can also notice

    that I am resting

    that's right

I am resting deeper

    and more calmly now

with every passing word

and every gentle breath

breathing gently...

gently breathing

    that's right

I am resting and reading effortlessly

    and noticing

that I can imagine the pillow

beneath my head

feels comfortable and relaxed

deeper

and with every easy

    effortless word

I can continue to imagine

noticing the feeling of the sheets

against my skin

and this feels comforting

    that's right

relaxing

deeper

with every word

blinking softly

that's right

and noticing that any sensation that I have

is just a sensation

effortlessly passing

and I say to myself…

"there's a sensation

        and here I am resting"

that's it

"and it feels so good

        to be in bed resting"

"the pillow feels comforting"

        "and the sheets feel warm"

as I relax

deeper now

and rest with confidence

I can notice now

that thoughts come and go

like clouds in the sky

or champagne bubbles rising

    resting a moment

    and popping

        that's right

I can say to myself

"there's a thought

    and here I am resting"

"and the pillow feels nice"

    that's it

"and the sheets feel comforting"

"and there's a sound

and here I am

    resting deeper now..."

ever so easily

relaxing into my deepest

    relaxation

and noticing that thoughts ...

    and sounds

come...

    and

        go

with every gentle breath

I do not mind noticing them

    as they drift by

I feel restfulness increasing now

relaxing deeper

deeper relaxing

with ease

I can imagine how good it will feel

    to wake up refreshed

while thoughts come and go

        rise and pop

as I notice that I am resting

and relaxing

    ever deeper now

noticing the pillow and the sheets

and even the thoughts and sounds

and the occasional sensations

        that come and go

means I can continue to relax

and rest

deeper now

naturally now

that's right.

Chapter 7

Lifestyle Considerations for Better Sleep

Of course there are so many factors that can and do influence sleep and sleeplessness. Through my own past experience of sleeplessness and also with respect to the many clients I have worked with, I have noticed that there are lifestyle influences that continue to show up.

By no means is this the definitive list, and I am sure that I have missed quite a few. Having said that, if sleeplessness has been a challenge and you are prepared to consider and/or make even a few of these lifestyle changes, then surprises are on their way to you.

General Health

There is no separation between mind and body. Modern medical science, psycho-neuro-immunology and alternative medicine are demonstrating that thoughts and feelings can influence and generate health or illness.

We are generally aware that our physical health has an influence on our thoughts and feelings and yet no matter which way round we look at this intricate flow of energy, sleeplessness is often a first sign that something is out of balance in our health and lifestyle.

Consider the state of your health and if you have questions about your health see a health practitioner. This is obvious and yet so many people live their lives completely oblivious to the fact that they have compromised health.

Our general state of health is a reflection of the inner workings of mind and emotions, and yet most people are only aware of how they physically `feel, not the thinking or the emotions that caused the feelings.

Working with a health practitioner while changing the patterns of sleep will enhance the process and enable the body/mind to make the changes it needs to make.

Taking your general health into consideration will also allow you to acknowledge that the body is designed to heal when it is resting and that some sleeplessness can be caused by an active body attempting to heal.

Solution:

- Take an honest look at your health and lifestyle choices. Consider that your health is indeed a reflection of your moment-to-moment thoughts and feelings.

- Talk to a health professional if you have any questions about your health.

- Consider your body as an intelligent and curious extension of your mind. One of the best forms of health re-balancing is mental awareness.

~ // ~

Stress

Without doubt, stress and specifically work and money-related stress is a persistent and often debilitating aspect of modern living, and yet stress is primarily a product of interpretation. Our history and beliefs will influence how we respond to the events of our day. Our response is what will either generate stress or not.

The stress that we carry in our mind/body will have a direct bearing on our ability to relax and of course to sleep. Practicing EFT, Self-Hypnosis and also creating 'space' for yourself will have a profound and positive influence on your life and perception of events.

Practicing 'napping' or 'power napping' has been demonstrated to reduce stress and also reduce the amount of sleep required at night. Refer to appendix for suggestions on creating your own 'power napping' session.

Meditation is universally recognised as an effective tool for reducing stress and generating mental states of calm.

Solution:

- Consider that your stress levels are a response to your 'perception' of events. Check how you are seeing the world, how your are responding 'inside' to the ever changing world and ask: *"Does my response serve me?"* or *"is this the only truth?"* or *"what if I thought about it another way?"*

- Be easy on yourself. You cannot know what you don't know. Most of your responses are learned, so check 'inside' yourself for a moment and ask… "is there another way, - can I do things differently here?"

- Make meditation a daily practice. Investigate Transcendental Meditation, Vipassana Meditation, Shri Chimnoy, Zen Buddhism for example.

- Set aside time to Power-Nap. Listen to relaxing or trance inducing music.

- Make space for yourself - time-out. Some of the most potent learnings we gain happen when we are resting or simply 'away' from stress.

~ // ~

Evening Meal

A very powerful piece of advice I was given that continues to be a 'winner' for my clients is Eat Light at Night.

Getting into bed with a heavy, full stomach means the digestion will be working very hard most of the night. This effort will take energy away from the body's healing, rebuilding and rejuvenation processes. A heavy, full stomach can mean the body may not be able to relax into a natural rhythm of dream (REM) sleep and deep sleep. It may also cause us to wake up feeling unrested.

Many clients have found that changing from red to white meat and including more salads or green vegetables at night has a very positive influence on sleep processes.

Another consideration at night is the <u>focus</u> on eating. Do you watch TV while you eat? When we watch TV and eat we are in a non-food focused state of mind which generally means we do not have any consciousness of what we are eating. The stomach does not get the initial messages from the sight of food to know what is coming. This is why it is so easy to overeat while in front of the box.

Interestingly, Yale studies showed that adults eat more and continue to eat more because of TV advertising between shows, which is great for the advertisers and yet not good for your sleep or your health.[3]

Solution:

- Check your evening meal. How much are you eating and is the food easy to digest or requiring more work?

---

[3] Priming Effects of Television Food Advertising on Eating Behavior.
Jennifer L. Harris, John A. Bargh, and Kelly D. Brownell
Yale University

- Look for alternative foods that are satisfying and yet lighter, less dense and yet enjoyable.

- Eat at the table not in front of TV. Talk to each other and eat slowly with your attention on the taste of the food.

- Talk to a health professional who understands food and how it can help you to take control of your sleeping patterns.

$$\sim // \sim$$

Stimulants

Coffee, tea, drugs, anything that can influence our mental and physical state and cause arousal need to be cut back. It's a no-brainer and yet sometimes we just don't consider the obvious.

Solution:

- Release stimulant use up to 4 hours before bedtime.

- Stop coffee intake after 2pm.

- Look for alternatives to the coffees and teas etc. There are many refreshing, and delicious alternatives available.

- If you are experiencing an addiction, talk to someone who can help. Hypnotherapy and NLP are powerful addiction releasing tools. Also, there are so many agencies and health practitioners that can give you tools to make a change.

~ // ~

Medication

If you are on medication for an illness or indeed for sleep, you may need to consult your health professional for an update on any possible side effects.

Sometimes my clients have realised that the combination of medications, rather than one medication alone has caused side effects that interfere with sleep.

Solution:

- Talk to your health professional about your medication and also consult a natural health professional for alternative possibilities.

- Look at all possibilities - conventional and non-conventional for your medication requirements. Remember medical science is only a few hundred years old while Chinese medicine for example is 5000 years old. Wisdom comes with time.

~ // ~

Get to bed by Ten

Grandma's advice: "One hour of sleep before midnight is worth 2 hours after"

I believe this is one of the most powerful and health re-building changes that you can make to your daily sleep routine. This simple change in routine was a life-saving strategy for me. This adjustment alone, during many years of illness and insomnia gave me the foothold that I needed to rebuild my sleep and health. It didn't sort the problem out and yet this simple change was revolutionary.

This is a big one for many. I have heard too many people with sleeping issues describe the same scenario: *"Because I sleep so badly I stay up until I am really tired"*, or *"If I don't get to sleep I just get up and watch TV or read a book"*.

Question: Do you notice that around 11pm at night you are getting your 'second wind'?

This 'second wind' is because your metabolic system is waking up to cleanse, rebuild and re-balance your body. The metabolic system wakes up while you are asleep and processes toxins, rebuilds cells, integrates new information and more. This is called 'Pitta' time in Ayurveda - traditional Indian medicine.

If you are awake at this time, your mind will become more alert and active simply because your body has lifted its game so that it can do this very important job.

In Ayurveda – an ancient Indian healing science – there are three specific time periods of the day relating to body vibration and rhythm:

- Pitta (fire) 10 – 2 am/pm
- Vata (air/space) 2 – 6 am/pm
- Kapha (earth/water) 6 – 10 am/pm

The fire time is when digestion is generally at its peak. Get to bed before 10pm and that means your head is on the pillow before the heating cycle begins. Generally you will drop into sleep at this time especially when you use the *Better Sleep Sooner* strategies.

~ // ~

Witching hour

If you notice you wake up between 2 and 6 am, this is the air/space time. At this time of the sleep cycle your sleep may be quite shallow and dreamy and so the ability to wake up easily or to be awoken easily is increased. This time is often called the 'witching hour' because it is a 'trance like' time. A fantastic time of the day for casting spells or meditating.

Solution:

- Check the time you are getting to bed and consider that it may not be in accordance with natural bodily or 'nature's' rhythms.

- Commit to getting into bed by 10pm for 2 weeks. You can always go back to the other habit and yet try this new time out and notice what happens.

- Become curious about the patterns of your body and how they work in harmony with nature. Understanding the *'witching hour'* for example can help you to relax a little when you wake up in the night. Recognising the 'second-wind' effect can give you an insight to how important it is to get to bed a little earlier.

~ // ~

Exercise

What exercise are you taking? When do you exercise and for how long?

Exercise has too many psycho-biological benefits to list and activates so many positive and curative systems within our bodies, one of which (when done in moderation) is the release of stress and tension.

On a daily basis I practice the Tibetan 5 Rites. An ancient and recently revived form of exercise that has only five general movements. Similar to Asana practice in yoga which I have also practiced for over 20 years, the 'Rites' exercise and massage most of the body and yet can be completed in less than 20 minutes.

Stretching is also an essential activity for creating a healthy and flexible body. Flexibility in body can be a reflection of flexibility of mind. Good flexibility can give the body/mind more freedom and scope to relax in bed. When we are well-exercised and flexible our body is more able to release stress and tension.

Solution:

- Increase your exercise and flexibility as a compliment to healthy living, stress relief and sleep.

- Investigate alternative exercise and stretching ideas like yoga for example.

- Find a friend who will commit to a routine with you or find a group that you can join.

- Walk. Walking alone has too many benefits to mention and it is an exercise that you can do anywhere and with very little preparation or gear.

$$\sim // \sim$$

Media

It is said that the brain has to increase functioning in order to interpret TV and the fast movement of the TV signal. This is why it is so easy to drift into a 'daze' or trance state while watching TV, simply because the mind has to change its vibrational state in order to make sense of the information coming from the TV.

Today's TV shows run at a much faster rate than 20 years ago, so generally we have to work harder to keep up. Also the content of late night or mid-evening TV is very different to what it was 20 years ago, so our minds can be more affected by the graphic or morbid nature of the programming.

I say programming with caution and yet with reason. There is a way to induce hypnosis when working with a client, and this involves two specific processes:

I. bypass the critical factor of the mind

II. create selective focus or attention

Let me explain:

1. TV bypasses the critical (or criticising) aspect of the conscious mind simply because we simply 'switch off' consciously when we watch a fictional program. We stop questioning the validity or reality, we simply go along for the ride .

2. TV acts as a focal point. A point where we have selective focus. Once we are entranced by the TV program, it is sometimes difficult to pull ourselves away.

These two factors are the start points for hypnotic induction and so when we sit down to a session of TV programs, we are really sitting down to a session of trance induced 'programming'.

Sally's Story

Sally came to me because she was not only having trouble sleeping, she was having bizarre and often violent dreams. Sally was not sleeping at all well.

I asked her what her TV habits were and where her TV was located in the house. Sally would watch TV in bed and would watch the detective, or murder investigation type programs and then switch off the light and try to go to sleep.

I suggested to Sally that she remove the TV from the bedroom and to turn the TV off half an hour before bed. I also suggested that if she had to watch those programs, maybe she could record them and watch them during the day.

Sally was watching brain-stimulating, trance-inducing TV in the place of rest and sleep while in a hypnotic state. The programs were about murder, mystery and people with psychological imbalances. Very compelling.

Bring these factors together and you have an outcome that is subconscious dis-harmony. Falling asleep or at least lying in bed trying to sleep with all that 'programming' in the brain would be very unsettling.

Sally changed her nightly ritual slowly and yet reported that after a few weeks of progressive 'withdrawal', she was getting to bed earlier and sleeping without disturbance.

Solution:

- Remove the TV, laptop, tablet, phone and any stimulating media from the bedroom. The bedroom is a place of respite, rest, self care and calm.

- Stop watching TV ½ an hour before bed so the mind and body can settle down and relax into rest.

- If you have to do something, have a bath, read a book, have a chat, take a short gentle walk, write a poem etc, and yet do it away from bed.

- Turn the internet off an hour or so before bed. The screen is blaring at you and unlike a TV you are much closer. Internet is constant and it is interactive and highly stimulating.

- Try something different... surprise yourself.

$$\sim // \sim$$

Trauma

Life and sleep can be turned upside down by a trauma. Trauma can create biological shifts in the body that we are often consciously unaware of. These shifts can create imbalances that over time influence our mental and physical health.

How do we deal with trauma? Well, generally we just have to 'get over it' and carry on because life carries on. This old 'soldier on' paradigm however, is being challenged. In modern research into health and disease, the 'soldier on' attitude is showing itself to be less than useful.

An unresolved trauma if unchecked can continue to influence the mind and body for months or even years, and it may only be through a physical (or mental) illness, or sleeplessness that we become aware of the influence of this trauma.

Solution:

- If your sleeplessness is not correcting itself using the techniques and strategies in this book, then it may be persisting because there is an event or trauma in the memory that is unresolved.

- Consider that with a little courage you can release these 'past' emotions with good, professional coaching.

- Timeline Therapy, NLP and Hypnotherapy can literally dissolve trauma from the past and without the need to relive it. Believe it or not, with NLP and Timeline therapy, you don't even have to talk about the trauma - what Self-Hypnosis and EFT to help you to release unwanted emotions from a trauma.

- Be honest with yourself, and treat any coaching that you may choose to get as an opportunity for self discovery and of course a *Better Sleep Sooner*.

~ // ~

Depression

"At least 80% of depressed people experience insomnia", - Psychology Today.

It is true that excessive sleeplessness can lead to depression, and yet another symptom of depression is over-sleeping. And after you get all of that under your belt, it is probably a good idea to just acknowledge how you are feeling from moment-to-moment. Honour your experience and with a little courage talk to someone who will listen and who also has some useful tools to move you forward.

Depression is a debilitating experience and unless checked can take over our thoughts, feelings, decisions and our life. As I stated in the beginning of this book, sleeplessness is a behaviour and as a behaviour it is something we can change. Depression is no different. Depression is something we are 'doing' and that means it can be altered and in some cases - 'undone'.

Solution:

• Take a moment and gather your courage then pick up the phone and talk to someone.

• Depression, I believe, is not an illness, it is a subconscious behaviour. It is the way the mind is choosing to experience life based upon perceptions of the past. More often than not, healing the past can release depression.

  • **Look up**. It is physiologically and neurologically difficult to feel depressed when you look up. Weird and yet for many - a life-saver. So, when you are feeling a little down... **Look up!**

  • See a health professional. There are so many variables to depression and one way to make a difference may be found in your diet or lifestyle.

  • A tip from me. Don't watch the TV news or read the morning paper. It is hypnotic and generally unhappy or negative information.

~ // ~

Anxiety

Anxiety is characterised generally by looking into the future and anticipating an event going bad or looking into the future and anticipating negative feelings. Anxiety about getting to sleep is a major contributor to sleeplessness and yet it uses most of the same mental strategies that we use to get excited about a future event. The major difference between anxiety and excitement is:

- Excitement is looking into the future and <u>imagining ourselves</u> having a great time.

- Anxiety is to imagine <u>being</u> in the future having a bad time and feeling bad.

This would suggest that one of the most useful ways of overcoming anxiety is:

- If/when feeling anxious, notice that the anxiety is about a task of event in the future. Acknowledge this to yourself and then create a mindset of curiosity.

- Now imagine yourself calm and relaxed after this imagined task or event… see yourself <u>Calm and Happy</u>.

Anxiety is generally an 'associated' (in the body) and uncomfortable experience, while true excitement is generally a dissociated (seeing ourselves) experience.

In NLP there is an anti-anxiety strategy that goes like this: Imagine yourself 15 minutes after the <u>successful</u> completion of the upcoming event or task.

This strategy is similar to the one discussed earlier. Because anxiety is future based, it makes sense to run a strategy that creates a better future experience. And because anxiety is in our imagination, we may as well use our imagination to work with it and dissolve it.

So, when it comes to sleep, the strategy of imagining yourself 15 minutes after the successful completion of 'the sleep' is the best practice for overcoming anxiety about sleeping.

Note: this strategy is one that requires a little practice especially if you are an anxiety specialist. Practice it on mundane things like: imagine yourself in the future - having successfully completed the 'tooth-brushing' process.

Get into the habit of running this strategy and sooner than later your brain will notice that excitement is more fulfilling than anxiety.

Solution:

- Use the anti-anxiety strategy mentioned earlier.

- Commit to becoming more and more conscious of the interplay of your mind and how 'imaginings' effect your body.

- Play with the future – imagine fun, silly, ludicrously funny scenarios so that you can create flexibility in you mind.

- Learn to relax.

- Smile :-), it's all in your mind.

$$\sim // \sim$$

Belief

Is it difficult to believe that it is possible to change your sleep problem? Then you are probably right, at least until you ask yourself:

What if I <u>can</u> change this problem?

What if I <u>can</u> continue to learn and let nature do what it is designed to do?

What if this sleeplessness that I have been having, now means I am even more inspired to commit to this strategy?

Our beliefs define our reality, and where we focus our thoughts we create our reality. The beliefs we have are generally borrowed or pre-programmed, very seldom do we generate a belief of our own and that can often mean we will not give a new idea the space or time simply because it is not familiar – we do not believe it will work.

Beliefs continue over time only because we continue to fuel them. We continue to give them space, even when we know they are faulty or have out-served their purpose. And what is a belief? An opinion, idea, rule, or perception that has continued to be unchallenged over time.

Here's the challenge: change your beliefs and do it now. Start by imagining yourself experiencing the change you want simply because you trusted in yourself to do something different - something new. See yourself having woken up yet again from a fabulous sleep. Why not? -, you have nothing to lose.

Solution:

- Imagine a future time when you have been waking up from a deep sleep everyday for a month… then remember that you have healed cuts, maybe healed broken bones, learned to walk, talk, write and a million other things that are now automatic behaviours.

- Also consider that having any beliefs about it working or not is pointless when instead, you could simply decide to do it, regardless of belief. Simply commit to the process as you have done with so many new ideas or strategies and be surprised by what happens.

- Consider how much creative potential lives within you just waiting for a new and fascinating idea or direction.

20 Simple Tips for a *Better Sleep Sooner*

1. Set a routine that you can comfortably commit to for 30 days, that way you are giving yourself the time to create new Habits.

2. Create a ritual of some type so that the mind and body can 'attune' to the resting process before you get into bed. One example would be to imagine leaving your 'day' at the bedroom door as you enter your bedroom.

3. Make your bedroom a place that says 'Rest and relaxation'. Make your bedroom comforting and rest-inducing.

4. Be in bed by 10. This will enable your mind and body to re-align with the cycles of nature.

5. Make your bedroom the place of rest and intimacy, nothing else. Your mind and body flourish when there are clear boundaries.

6. Make sure the bedroom is dark. The eye can detect very small amounts of light. Even if you have an illuminated clock by the bed, cover it or remove it.

7. Remove all TV's, stereos, phones, laptops, portable devices or media-type devices from the bedroom, this will remove any possible mental distraction.

8. Do not read electronic devices in bed they produce light and stimulate the eyes and brain. Read these devices away from the bed.

9. A warm bath before bed can lift the temperature of the body so that when you get into bed the natural drop in body temperature will aid the process of drifting into sleep.

10. Eat light at night so that the body is not working so hard during the sleep period, which means your body and mind can relax deeper and rejuvenate properly.

11. Exercise early in the evening. This lifts the body temperature and also burns excess energy and stress so that you can relax and rest easily when you are in bed.

12. Power-nap, meditate or take short rest breaks during the day to release stress and tension.

13. Clarify the mental and physical state you want to be in tomorrow morning and picture it

clearly. Remember; when we know where we are going it is easier to get there.

14. If you wake up in the night to go to the bathroom, try to keep lights off or very dim. Any light that shines in the night can shut off melatonin (sleep chemicals in the body).

15. Avoid stimulants such as coffee before bed and also avoid alcohol as it interferes with the deep sleep and healing cycles of the body .

16. Reduce fluid intake before bed and that way you are less likely to have to go to the bathroom during the night.

17. Check your general health. For example being overweight can have a significant influence on your ability to sleep. Your health professional will be able to do this for you. It may be a lifesaver and a huge benefit to your sleep.

18. Get professional help if you need it. Sleep is an absolute must and any help to get you back into a healthy sleeping rhythm is time and money well spent.

19. Discuss any medication or herbal remedies that you may be taking with your health practitioner.

Temporary use of medication or herbs can get your sleep back on track.

20. Relax and rest... simply close your eyes and rest.

Chapter 8

Stoems for a *Better Sleep Sooner*

A little rest now, can mean a deeper sleep later.

Sleep is so important and so mysterious. Adding some time to relax during your day or at least taking time out to allow your mind and body to relax, just a little, can take the edge off the stress and tension that you may be taking to bed.

The stoems that follow are designed to help you to relax and to release any 'inner objections' to enjoying a *Better Sleep Sooner*. They are designed to be read slowly, so give yourself a little space and time to settle back and relax.

Self-Hypnosis Stoem
for healing sleeplessness

This stoem is designed to be read slowly and with complete attention so that these words are able to make suggestions to your subconscious mind while you read. It is designed specifically to address any possible underlying 'root cause' issues that may have been contributing to the sleeplessness in your past, which means...

I am effortlessly reading these words

move across

and

      down

the page
and that means
I can continue to relax
into a deeper calm

calmly relaxing

relaxing calmly

noticing that my breathing changes

as I continue to relax

    that's right

and I notice muscles relaxing
in certain parts of my body
becoming a little more

ever so gently
relaxing into reading

happens effortlessly

as I allow myself to let go
just enough

    that's right

with every gentle word
and each careful movement

of each confident word

may effortlessly inspire
my mind to be open
to positive and useful suggestions
designed for me to gently relax

Chapter 8   Better Sleep Sooner

relax gently

and learn effortlessly

effortlessly learning

as I continue to notice
I can feel confident in myself
to continue to read
and wonder
ever so curious

as if in a dream

        that's right

I can calm deeper down
ever so gently deeper

deeper gently
gently breathing

breathing gently

and blinking softly

softly blinking

                    that's right

and considering with ease
that the small change I make

within me now
can create a change
that influences my thoughts
and feelings
while dissolving sleeplessness

from my past
and future
as I read
and wonder how
I am *continuing* to heal
any past experience
that may have once caused sleeplessness
is a thing of the past
and behind me now

                    that's right

which means
I can feel more and more confident

to notice that
with each passing word

relaxing me deeper

and

deeper

I can notice
really notice

that any past sleeplessness
I may have once had
is healing itself now

as I read confidently and consider
with growing confidence
just how successfully
my mind and body continue to
heal and rebalance
those events of the past
release these emotions now

as easily as I breathe effortlessly
releasing

and trusting deeper
deeper trusting

which means
I am even more inspired to trust myself
and to notice
that because the past

 is healing itself

                now

      that's right

I can just relax

          and rest

a little deeper
which means
I can imagine myself
15 minutes after waking up
from a deep sleep

feeling relaxed and refreshed

refreshed and relaxed

and noticing more and more
how I can feel completely relaxed
and detached completely

from any past sleeplessness
is a thing of the past

and that means
I can picture myself
after waking from a deep sleep

because deep sleep

happens naturally
now that I can let go

and rest deeply

when in bed

simply rest

      resting simply

inviting sleepiness
occurs naturally
confidently noticing
that the more I think about sleep
the more I imagine resting
deeper and

deeper

that's it

feeling a growing confidence now
that I can continue to notice
that I am anticipating

feeling refreshed
and happy every morning
I wake up
feeling rejuvenated

and fully AWAKE NOW…

YES!

Relaxation Stoem

Sometimes
relaxation can occur effortlessly
while I am reading
and that means
I can continue to notice

relaxation increasing

as I read each comfortable word
reminds me to notice that my arms

    can relax
        and soften

    soften
        and relax

as I drift with each word

into an ever more dreamy
and comfortable state

of relaxation

is easy to invite
into every muscle
relaxing deeper

deeper relaxing

noticing and feeling

more and more aware

that when I relax
the challenges that I *was* having
seem to slip away

      that's right

into insignificance
as I continue to deepen
this gentle feeling

releasing any tension
noticing my breath

      coming

            and going

as I read and wonder
how deeply can I relax

while I read
and continue to feel
more and more comfortable now

that I notice that any sounds
simply drift into the distance

and that means I can focus
deeper and more confidently
as I recognise my natural

ability to relax

and to rebalance
is increasing now
with every gentle word

and every gentle breath
that comes and

    goes

just like any old tension
or confusion

    worries or concerns
simply dissolving behind me

like footprints in the sand

as if confidently walking

along a quiet
    beautiful beach

where every step I take now
means I am even more inspired

to notice opportunities to relax
and unwind

and rebalance

and refresh
my mind and body
are infinitely creative
and responsive now
to my intention to relax more
and a little deeper
regardless of where I am
or who I am with
I am inspired to notice
more and more
that I can feel calm
and relaxed

relaxed and calm

and more responsible now
for how I think and feel
that I can let go now

of old destructive patterns
      of the past
while unconsciously generating
new and exciting ways

that I can look after myself easily

which means
as I imagine walking

on a beautiful beach
that the ocean
powerful and relaxed

relaxed and powerful

is dissolving those footprints
behind me now

      effortlessly releasing

           releasing effortlessly

so that I can look forward
to the future
appears brighter now

which means I can move forward
with anticipation

I can picture myself
every morning

feeling wide awake

and

completely refreshed

and with every breath

and every word
I can continue to feel
that a change has been made

which means
I can notice wakeful energy
flowing into my body

so I can feel

more and more AWAKE

NOW!

Appendix

Better Sleep Sooner Self-Hypnosis

Notes for success with Self-Hypnosis

Self-Hypnosis is self-directed relaxation designed for you to take yourself into a relaxed and receptive state of mind and body. Your subconscious mind is more open and more likely to act upon suggestions that are made when you are relaxed and at ease.

This script is designed to be read into a recording device and then played back to yourself. When reading the script, take your time. Read with conviction. Pause for a moment at the '||pause||', and when you notice a word like relax, say it slowly and with a relaxed tone. Tone is everything. So give it a go, it's fun.

Outcome check

Before you begin a session of Self-Hypnosis make sure you have a clear outcome in mind. Be very clear why you are doing the Self-Hypnosis session. Picture yourself in the future 15 minutes after waking from another wonderful sleep - refreshed and energised.

Defining your outcome is probably the most essential aspect of any self-directed process. Be clear and committed to the outcome and that way your subconscious mind will respond well to the suggestions that you give it.

Self-Hypnosis Script

N.B. Read the following script into a recording device and then play it back to yourself.

Now that you have taken the time…

to look after yourself…

take a moment to settle back…

and to let your eyes close…

That's it…

||pause||

And with your eyes closed, I would like you to notice that you can imagine your eyelids are becoming more and more relaxed with every word I say...

more and more relaxed...

with every... gentle... breath...

that's it...

||pause||

and for a moment... I would like you to imagine that your eyes are sealed closed... completely sealed... your eyelids are becoming more and more relaxed and heavy... that's right... so heavy and relaxed that they just won't work...

and that means... you can just let go now...

and relax even deeper now...

that's it...

||pause||

letting go... a little more now... with every gentle breath...

that's it... just letting go...

relaxing and softening... softening and relaxing...

as the relaxation in your eyelids slides effortlessly into every muscle in your face... relaxing and letting go...

every muscle in your shoulders... relaxed and soft...

relaxation sliding down your spine... relaxing and softening... and into every muscle... relaxed and soft... every tendon... relaxed and at ease...

||pause||

And as you continue to relax... you can continue to consider the powerful changes you have already made to your ability to sleep...

that's right...

and how easily... you have made such lasting changes... changes that preserve themselves deep down inside so that you can continue to feel confident and relaxed about your ability to dissolve old habits so effortlessly...

that's right... so that you can relax and rest and feel confident about your ability to sleep...

||pause||

And you know that… you can… it's like you can relax a little deeper now… into your deepest relaxation… that's it… deeper now with every breath…

that's it…

you can easily imagine that you have been magically transported to a tropical island beach…

a long stretch of white sand… maybe you can feel the warmth of the sand beneath your feet… maybe a soft breeze caressing your skin… beautiful… crystal clear lagoon on one side… tropical rain forest on the other…

||pause||

and you are taking a gentle stroll along the beach… and with each confident step… relaxing deeper with every step…

knowing with absolute confidence that from now on you rest deeply every night… that's right… you do so effortlessly because now you know the secret… now you know how to rest deeply… relaxed and calm… calm and relaxed…

||pause||

you can imagine lying in bed and feeling that restful feeling… thoughts come and go in your mind, and you do not mind… you simply say "there's a thought… and here I am resting"… that's right…

||pause||

so easy to just relax now… now that you know that sleep is no longer an issue… sleep is no longer the goal… when you get into bed from now on you are on a relaxing and rejuvenating journey… the destination being that wonderful feeling of waking up refreshed and happy… that's right… you can imagine it now… as you take each confident and calming step along the beach… you can imagine now the feeling of complete fulfillment as you realise that you have just woken up from a deep and dream-filled sleep…

||pause||

You know how to do this… you now know the strategy and it is etched into your subconscious mind knows more than you think you know and that is like a dream… and with every step you notice that you are leaving footprints in the sand behind you… footprints of the old problems… the old worries and concerns now being swept away… that's it… old strategies dissolving with every effortless wave… and you wave good bye as waves of warm confidence flow through you and around you…

||pause||

You can now relax… no longer do the old stresses or concerns have any influence on your thoughts, feelings or behaviour… you are free now to choose your own path and feel excited and confident from now on… deep rest is your birthright and you now embrace this with confidence and certainty… and it feels fabulous… and continues to feel fabulous from this point forward…

||pause||

every step you take you feel lighter and more excited about your ability to rest deeply now… you trust that your body will take you naturally into sleep… and that means you can let go and enjoy your continued success as you step forward with confidence into your future…

||pause||

you can see yourself waking up each morning refreshed and revived… happy and refreshed… you can imagine the feeling of increased energy and confidence that comes with sleeping naturally now…

||pause||

that's right… from now on… when you are in bed… a thought is just a thought… "there's a thought…

and here I am resting…" a sound is simply a sound… "there's a sound… and here I am resting…" it's so easy to remember to relax now and just let go…

||pause||

and with every step you are now feeling as light as a feather… ready to bring all that you have learned... and this feeling of calm back into your day... lifting up and above this beautiful beach... free and in complete confidence as you return to this moment… listening easily and remembering all the things that continue to serve you every night from now on...

that's right...

||pause||

and in a moment I will count from 1 to 7...and you will easily wake yourself up from this deeply restful state… knowing on the number 7 your eyes will open… you will be refreshed and excited about your ability to rest deeply every night and to wake up every morning feeling refreshed and revived…

||pause||

one... slowly and easily coming back to full awareness…

||pause||

two… feeling energy and sensation coming back into fingers… toes… that's it

||pause||

three… knowing that the learnings and understandings have cemented themselves in now

||pause||

four… feeling more and more aware

||pause||

five… energy rising now

||pause||

six… your eyes have been cleansed in a cool clear spring and on the next number

||pause||

seven… wide awake…

Power-napping

Notes on success with your Power-nap

Your power-nap can be short and swift or a long luxurious dreamy experience. The strategies are the same regardless. The key is to know what you want from the nap. This is obvious, of course, and yet when I start a power-nap I am very clear about how long it will be and how I want to feel afterwards. This may seem crazy and yet, remember, your subconscious mind is waiting for compelling suggestions and your body is just waiting for your mind to set the course. So the clearer and the more compelling the suggestion, the better the experience and outcome.

How many times have you set the alarm and woken 2 minutes before it chimes? Your subconscious knows time and simply needs a clear instruction and a clear reason. After a while you will trust your subconscious ability to look after you and to wake you up when required, however, until that time occurs look at your watch if you are concerned about time. Looking at your watch will not have a negative influence on your nap... you will probably relax more.

How to run a Power-nap

Step One: Important consideration is 'where'. Choose a place where you will not be disturbed so that you can relax and let go completely. Turn the phone off, 'sleep' the computer, lock the door. It is necessary to make sure that your subconscious mind does not feel that it has to be alert for any disturbance.

Step Two: Define the duration of the nap. The length does not really matter, as long as you do it, you will gain benefits.

Step Three: Set the terms. "I will take a nap for 5 minutes and in that 5 minutes I will release stress and tension and re-energise myself so that when I wake up I feel great!"

Step Four: Picture yourself feeling great. Nice!

Memorise the next bit.

Step Five: Seated comfortably, close your eyes and soften your eyelids completely… that means imagine them becoming heavier and heavier, more and more relaxed, until you can imagine that they are sealed closed.

Step Six: Imagine you are stepping down 10 steps and with each step imagine becoming more and more relaxed… with every step say to yourself… "relaxing deeply… deeply relaxing"

Step Seven: Now imagine you are walking on a beach or in a beautiful relaxing place where you love to be. A place where you know you can relax deeply. Imagine that with every step you are relaxing more and that any stress or tension is simply dissolving away.

Step Eight: Allow your mind to drift and to wonder and when you notice that it has, simply bring yourself back to the beach and the walking.

Step Nine: When you know or feel that your time is up imagine the 10 steps in front of you and ascend the steps – counting from 1 to 10 to your self – knowing that when you get to the 10th step you will be wide awake and feeling great.

Smile.

Emotional Freedom Technique

Notes on success with EFT

EFT was developed by Gary Craig and was designed to release emotional blockages by tapping acupressure or meridian points on the face, upper body and hands.

Since the creation of EFT there have been many changes to the technique, the most interesting being the simplification of it.

I use EFT myself and I use it with clients in order to release and/or soften emotional energy. As I said earlier in the book, emotions are often the glue that hold habits, beliefs and motivations in place. Using EFT can help to dissolve the glue so that we can move on.

Using EFT can relax and de-clutter the mind so that when we are in bed resting, the mind can let go and drift into sleepy bliss. Try it and be surprised.

Outcome check

Forgive the repetition, however, before you begin a session of EFT make sure you have a clear outcome in mind. Be very clear why you are doing the EFT session.

The outcome could be: picture yourself in a future time, 15 minutes after waking from another wonderful sleep - refreshed and energised. See yourself feeling refreshed and energised and make the image compelling.

The EFT Technique

The diagram (opposite) comes from the original EFT technique. Each point is tapped with the tips of 1st and 2nd fingers about 7 times.

The basic structure of an EFT session is:

Calibrate → Tap → Calibrate ? → Exit

repeat ↵

Calibrating your emotional state before and after each round is an essential part of the EFT strategy. It will give you constant feedback with regards to your progress.

Tapping Points

- top of head
- eyebrow
- side of eye
- under eye
- under nose
- under lip
- collarbone
- under arm (4 in.)
- karate chop

EFT Routine

The basic EFT routine is as follows and in this routine we are working on Anxiety about Sleep.

Step one: *Calibration*

Scale the intensity of the issue you are addressing from 0 - 10

How strong is the feeling of anxiety? 0 being the least. (0 = not an issue, or no discomfort & 10 = a major issue, or strong discomfort)

Step Two: *Set up Statement*

Begin Tapping the 'karate chop' point on one hand while repeating the setup statement. This may go like, "Even though I feel this anxiety, I deeply and completely accept myself" or "Even though I have this anxiety, I love and accept myself completely".

Say the setup phrase just a few times while repeatedly tapping the karate point.

Step Three: *Reminder Statement Tapping Sequence*

Have a memory or thought of an anxious moment about sleep in the back of your mind while doing the next step.

We begin to do what is called a 'round' of tapping. At this stage we are tapping the negative emotion and the negative emotion is a described by the 'reminder phrase'. e.g.. "This feeling of anxiety"

Beginning at the eyebrow point we tap each point 7 times in the following order while repeating the reminder phrase.

1. Eyebrow "this feeling of anxiety"
2. Side of eye "this anxiety about sleep"
3. Under eye "this feeling of anxiety"
4. Under nose "I feel anxious about sleep"
5. Chin "feeling anxious"
6. Collarbone "anxiety"
7. Under arm "I feel so anxious"
8. Head "feeling anxious"

As you move from point to point, be aware that other thoughts or feelings may come up for you. This is a sign that you are releasing surface emotions and exploring deeper feelings - and so <u>follow</u> the new emotions as they come up and keep tapping. If you notice that you are feeling more nervous than anxious, say "this nervous feeling".

At times it is also good to repeat the 'setup statement' while continuing your tapping round, e.g., "even thought I have this anxiety I love and forgive myself completely"

Complete three rounds and then re-calibrate, 0-10 to notice how you are feeling now. Change can often happen in the first few rounds so really notice the difference in the way you now feel, and if you are still self-calibrating above zero, continue to tap.

Step Four: *Positive Tapping Sequence*

This is the point where we begin to tap for the positive programming. Positive feelings and thoughts, ideas and directions we wish to go instead of the negative direction.

Tapping the same points as in step three, we begin at the eyebrow…

1. Eyebrow "I choose to release this old feeling now"
2. Side of eye "I choose to trust myself"
3. Under eye "Relaxed and calm in bed"
4. Under nose "Listening to my intuition"
5. Chin "Happiness"
6. Collarbone "I choose to be calm"
7. Under arm "Inner peace"
8. Head "Feelings of freedom"

The next round can be different again.

1. Eyebrow "Even though I used to feel anxious"
2. Side of eye "I know I can take control now"
3. Under eye "I choose to feel happy "
4. Under nose "I choose to be good to myself"
5. Chin "Happiness and fulfillment"
6. Collarbone "Excited about the future"
7. Under arm "Inner peace"
8. Head "Feelings of happiness"

After two positive rounds it is time to re-calibrate how you are feeling about the original issue. Where on the scale of 0 - 10 does it sit now?

If the issue still has a degree of discomfort - continue the process.

For best results:

1. Define your outcome
2. Repeat, repeat, repeat
3. Be honest with yourself

Visit the official EFT website www.emofree.com for more information, free downloads and a phenomenal resource for testimonials and articles.

Better Sleep Sooner Strategy - Quick Reference

Have a clear image of yourself in the morning 15 minutes after waking up - feeling refreshed and happy.

When you get into bed notice that you *are* <u>resting</u> and repeat the following to yourself as internal dialogue when lying in bed.

★ *"It is so good to be in bed... resting"*

★ *"Here I am resting... the sheets feel wonderful"*

★ *"Here I am resting... and the pillow feels nice"*

When you notice thoughts

★ *"There's a thought - <u>and</u> here I am resting"*

When you notice sounds

★ *"Ah... there's a sound - <u>and</u> here I am resting"*

When you notice sensations

★ *"Ah...there's a sensation... <u>and</u> I am resting"*

Other Publications by Aaron McLoughlin

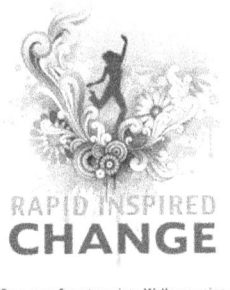

Rapid Inspired Change. Turn your Symptoms into Wellbeing using The Fascination Principle.

Available online through www.rapidinspiredchange.com

Consultations with Aaron McLoughlin in Byron Bay, and the Gold Coast, Australia, or by Skype.

Check http://www.bettersleepsooner.com for more details.

www.ingramcontent.com/pod-product-compliance
Lightning Source LLC
Chambersburg PA
CBHW071426160426
43195CB00013B/1829